Helping Children Manage Anxiety at School

A Guide For Parents and Educators In Supporting The Positive Mental Health of Children in Schools

BY

COLLEEN WILDENHAUS

D1157200

This book is dedicated to

Julia, who shows anxiety that SHE is in charge every day.

Ryan, your kindness and compassion make the world a better place.

Richie, your love and support are what most spouses only dream of, yet I get to live it.

And...thank you for the computer!

Table of Contents

For Educators:

"Everyone is a genius. But if you judge a fish by its ability to climb a tree, it will live its whole life believing it is stupid."- Albert Einstein

For Parents:

"Parenthood is about raising and celebrating the child you have, not the child you thought you would have. It's about understanding that they are exactly the person they are supposed to be and that, if you're lucky, they just might be the teacher who turns you into the person you are supposed to be." ~ Joan Ryan

For Children:

"You are braver than you believe, stronger than you seem, and smarter than you think."- Christopher Robin

Introduction

Educators and parents play a pivotal role in helping a child cope with and manage anxiety while at school. This guide provides a foundational understanding of anxiety followed by practical steps in creating a classroom environment and individualized plans to support the anxious child. It highlights the critical role of educators, parents, and outside therapists (when applicable) in an anxious child's life.

As an educator since 2004, I have seen it all.

The girl hiding behind the drinking fountain worried about her goldfish dying.

The boy refusing to walk outside because he may encounter a bug.

The child crying for hours each morning, finally settling down at lunchtime.

The girl who never spoke in class or one on one with me.

The boy who refuses to take spelling tests each week.

The boy who replied to questions with an inappropriate response.

The girl who is afraid to come to school in case the fire alarm goes off.

The boy who keeps his head down nearly all day.

As a parent since 2005, I have raised a daughter with debilitating anxiety for most of her life. Today, through intense therapy and the necessary support at school, she is thriving. However, I will never forget...

My daughter's pleas to stay home from school.

The months and years that she did not attend classes.

Her tears as she begged me to help her be "normal" and have friends.

Hearing educators dismiss her anxiety as misbehavior.

Being told that I am an overprotective mother rather than her advocate.

Seeing her struggle academically from so much missed class time.

Having to quit a job that I loved in order to get her the help she deserved.

Do any of these scenarios sound familiar? If so, this book is for you. All of these situations showcase examples of anxiety in the classroom. There is definitely an appropriate and inappropriate way to respond. The inappropriate way leads to increased anxiety and feelings of despair while the appropriate way supports a child leading to happiness, independence, and confidence. Read on to discover the information you need to know in order to help anxious children manage their anxiety and thrive in the classroom.

Early on in my teaching, I spent an incredible amount of time trying various behavior management systems, all with the goal that the children would meet the classroom expectations presented to them. Never once did I realize I should look below the surface, and try to understand **why** the undesirable behaviors were occurring. Throughout my extensive educational training, the topic of "why" behaviors were occurring was never presented. The focus was on simply stopping the unwanted behaviors through rewards and/or punishment rather than on finding the source of the unwanted behaviors in order to teach the missing skills. I learned the red, yellow, and green system for behavior with the goal being to reward those students who met the expectations with an extra recess or a prize from the treasure chest, but I never learned that children who are making poor choices may be acting this way out of something other than choice. When a child wants to meet the expectations set by the teacher but is unable to because of anxiety, he loses motivation to work hard and succeed. This loss in motivation fuels anxiety, creating a negative, habitual cycle.

Once my daughter was born and we realized that we were raising a child with severe anxiety and OCD a switch clicked and suddenly, I looked back at individual children from my classroom and realized that I failed them each and every time they needed me. I treated their

4

behavior with a simple "you are misbehaving" philosophy. I now realize that child A was hitting because he couldn't express his anxious feelings during lunch or that child B was refusing to do writing because she was too worried about failing. Had I known then what I know now, I would have been able to pull out the root cause (anxiety), work through it, and over time see success in their unwanted behaviors. You now have the opportunity to teach these children in the way that they deserve with this clearly laid out guide.

How To Use This Book

While this book is slightly more geared for educators, it is just as useful for parents seeking ways to help a child at school as they work closely with schools to provide the needed support. This book specifically focuses on anxiety, while promoting ways to support the mental health of all children within the classroom. This guide is intended to be used by educators, parents, and therapists to gain an understanding of how anxiety affects children in the classroom, create a plan for managing anxiety in the classroom, and create and implement 504s or IEPs as needed. When this information is understood and followed with consistency, authenticity, and validity, children gain independence and confidence academically and mentally.

Educators, plan to read through the entire book, completing the exercises as they are shown throughout the chapters, and collect data when requested, prior to discussing or implementing any type of plan. Once you have finished reading the book in its entirety, completed the exercises, and collected the data, go back through step by step and begin creating a classroom atmosphere that supports the mental health of all children, specifically targeting children with anxiety as needed.

Parents, you should also plan to read the entire book before meeting with the school or devising a plan for your child. While the exercises are intended to be used by educators, you will benefit from many of the exercises as well, by simply changing the viewpoint to one in which you can relate. Your goal is to understand the ways in which you can help your child succeed at school. Depending on your child's school, you may need to use all of the information in this guide to educate the school on best practices for helping your child.

All of the exercises and images referenced throughout the book are available as a PDF download for those who purchase the book. The link for the downloadable PDFs can be found in the resource section at the end of the book. I suggest you print out the PDF versions to use for the exercises in this guide rather than using the ones within the text. There are over 20 additional "bonus" worksheets specifically created for educators, parents, and children to understand, acknowledge, and manage anxiety. These bonus worksheets are beneficial for all children (grade school through teens) and can be used for anxieties seen at school and at home.

At the completion of this book, educators and parents will have a solid understanding of how anxiety works, how it presents itself in the classroom, and the ways in which schools can support the mental health of all children, especially those with anxiety. (Many of the ideas centered on classroom anxiety can easily be applied to anxiety seen at home as well.) You will learn how to create classrooms with:

Strong educator-child relationships

Calm classroom environments

Normalization of anxiety

Positive language and tone

Improved problem-solving skills and emotional intelligence

Focus on effort over outcome

It should be noted, the term child is used rather than the word student throughout this book. "Student" refers to the child as he or she relates to school, where "child" refers to the whole of the person. "Child" will be used as the term for all ages of children within the school (preschool-high school). Similarly, the pronouns "he" and "she" will be used interchangeably throughout the text.

The plan outlined in this book can be used for children of all ages, preschool through high school. Of course, you will need to adjust your language and plan based on a child's age, but the premise is the same for everyone.

CHAPTER 1

Educate Yourself About Anxiety

As an educator, you wear many hats. It can be overwhelming to think of the responsibilities you have each day within your classroom, in addition to teaching the lessons you have prepared. You are a nurse, counselor, mediator, engineer, musician, artist, surrogate parent, cheerleader, and events coordinator. Do not worry. This plan does not add more to your already overflowing plate. It will actually streamline issues you are already juggling.

It is not your job to diagnose and label a child, but it is your job to be aware of signs of anxiety and to help implement anxiety management skills in order to reach every child to the best of your ability. For children with a current IEP or 504 plan related to anxiety, it is important that you monitor the plans for effectiveness. For children with less severe anxiety, you are responsible for helping them manage their anxiety in order to be successful in school. Most of the children who enter your classroom will be considered "typical", meaning they are able to be taught with a traditional, whole group style where few individual accommodations are necessary. However, there are children who enter your classroom that need extra TLC. Yes, these children may take extra time and patience, but every child is worth it. No child should ever be punished or fail academically due to anxiety.

A useful feature of this guide is that most of the ideas and suggestions can be applied to the entire class creating an atmosphere that promotes positive mental health for everyone. All children will benefit from improved strong teacher-child relationships, a calm classroom environment, the normalization of anxiety, positive language and tone, improved problem-solving skills and emotional intelligence, and focusing on effort over results. Of course, there will be individual needs that should be met outside of the whole class, but they will be minimal once you begin to understand how to create a classroom in which all personalities are addressed. You will notice a significant decrease in challenging behaviors among children by following the information presented throughout this book.

Prevalence of Anxiety in Children

Enthusiastic educators eagerly attend Professional Development opportunities, taking notes, listening attentively, and picturing ways to implement these new ideas in their classroom. Then reality hits and there is never enough time to get to the changes you want to make so you continue on the same path because it is working, but you know it could be better. I beg you to take the time to read this book, think of why you entered this profession (it wasn't for the pay), and then think of children who can benefit greatly from your understanding and implementation of what is offered in this book.

Children with anxiety deserve to come to school without the physical and mental weight, caused by excessive anxiety, that they carry around. They deserve to thrive socially and academically. Anxious children do not like the way that anxiety makes them feel. They want to be happy and confident.

Exercise 1: Before continuing, what do you already believe about anxiety...positive or negative?. What is your attitude towards anxiety? Be honest with yourself. Nobody will see this. Take a few moments to complete exercise 1. (Remember, these exercises can be printed as a PDF from the link provided in the resources section of the book.)

Exercise 1 focuses on understanding your thoughts about anxiety
PRIOR to reading this guide.

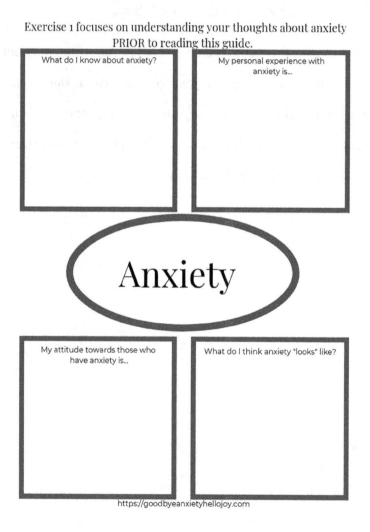

What do I know about anxiety?

My personal experience with anxiety is...

Anxiety

My attitude towards those who have anxiety is...

What do I think anxiety "looks" like?

https://goodbyeanxietyhellojoy.com

Have you ever felt anxious...the feeling of sweaty palms, lightheadedness, and a stomach full of butterflies? Do you feel this frequently throughout the day in a variety of situations or just when you fly in a plane or stand near the edge of a tall cliff? Anxiety is a normal feeling that everyone feels from time to time, but becomes a disorder when a child regularly feels disproportionate levels of it. If you have experienced the feeling of anxiety you may relate well to these anxious children in your class, but you may not know what to do to help them. If you do not experience regular anxiety (lucky you), then it can be really hard for you to understand and relate to their issues. Imagine your worst fear. Are you scared of snakes, small places, the dentist, or something happening to your loved ones?

Let's take snakes. Each day, you arrive at work and find that your classroom is full of non-venomous snakes. You must enter the classroom and perform your job as an educator while snakes slither around your feet. You are expected to follow your schedule, focus on teaching the plans you have created, patiently meet the needs of the children in your class, and keep everyone safe and engaged for the full school day. Pretty hard to imagine being your best self while knowing that your biggest fear is all around you for hours at a time.

This is what many kids deal with each and every day in the classroom. Of course, it may not be snakes. It may be the fear of germs, their safety in the wake of school shooting coverage, fearing the safety of their parents while they are away, the thought of making a mistake, the discomfort of having to be around other people, and so on.

Exercise 2: Think about your biggest fear. How do you react and respond when these events or thoughts occur. Brainstorm using exercise 2.

Exercise 2

My Biggest Fear

My biggest fear is...

When I encounter (or think about encountering) my biggest fear...what happens?

To My Mind...	To My Body...

How to you react or respond?

My response is...

Is it helpful? Why or why not?

https://goodbyeanxietyhellojoy.com

14

According to the *Journal of Developmental & Behavioral Pediatrics*[1] nearly 6 million American children suffer from anxiety. Of those children, 2.6 million have a diagnosed anxiety/depression disorder. That means that 1 in 8 school-aged children have a diagnosable anxiety disorder, while many others suffer from undiagnosed anxiety. Of the children with anxiety, up to 5% suffer from school refusal, meaning the anxiety is so high that the child refuses to go to school on a regular basis. Sadly, nearly 80% of children with diagnosable anxiety are not receiving any type of treatment according to the Anxiety and Depression Association of America, even though it is the most treatable mental health illness[2]. Untreated anxiety is the biggest indicator of depression later in life. Unfortunately, these numbers continue to rise each year. These statistics make it clear that every classroom has children suffering from anxiety. With or without the label of a disorder, anxiety can wreak havoc on a child academically, emotionally, mentally, and physically.

---

[1] https://www.cdc.gov/childrensmentalhealth/features/anxiety-and-depression.html
[2] https://adaa.org/about-adaa/press-room/facts-statistics

Exercise 3: Think about past and present children in your class. Do you think any child struggles/struggled with anxiety? If so, what makes you think this? Use exercise 3 to collect your thoughts.

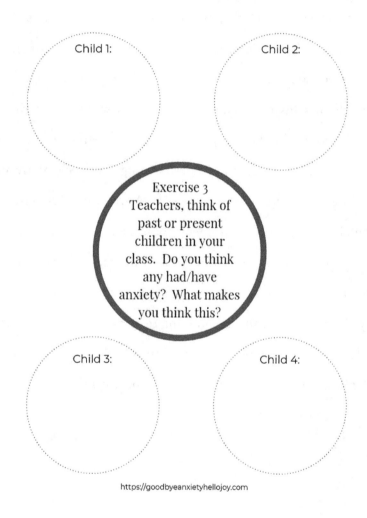

Child 1:

Child 2:

Exercise 3
Teachers, think of past or present children in your class. Do you think any had/have anxiety? What makes you think this?

Child 3:

Child 4:

https://goodbyeanxietyhellojoy.com

If you are a veteran educator, you may be thinking back over the years, wondering why it has only been in recent years that you have been noticing signs of anxiety in children. Since 2007, the rate of anxiety in kids and teens has continually risen[3]. This is due to a number of factors, including social media, technology, school safety, decrease in play for children, a shift in parenting trends, and increased academic pressures[4]. Regardless of the reason for the increase in anxiety, educators at all grade levels will be expected to teach children dealing with anxiety in their classroom.

In America, on average, children spend 180 days in school each academic year. Each day is roughly 7 hours, meaning that they spend 1,260 hours each year attending school. For children with anxiety, these 7 hours each day are exhausting, as they fight the anxiety every day, all day. Educators play an integral role in their anxiety management due to the vast amount of time children are in their care. As you will see, in order for anxiety to be managed, children of all ages must have supportive adults in their life following a consistent plan. If anxiety is only supported at home, and not during the 7 hours each day that the child is in school, it becomes increasingly difficult to successfully manage the anxiety and succeed in and out of school. In

---

[3] https://www.cdc.gov/childrensmentalhealth/data.html

[4] https://www.psychologytoday.com/us/blog/liking-the-child-you-love/201601/the-rising-epidemic-anxiety-in-children-and-teens

order for anxiety management to be successful, essential collaboration must occur between educators, parents, and outside therapists.

What is Anxiety?

It is natural for everyone to worry about things from time to time. What educator isn't a bit anxious on the first day of school, when being evaluated by the administration, making a challenging phone call to parents, or being asked to speak in front of others. You worry about your abilities, new situations and tasks, and making a mistake. However, most people can acknowledge what they are feeling and handle the situation properly. For children (and adults) with anxiety, the worries become all-encompassing because they do not have the knowledge or ability to handle situations, both real or perceived as real.

So, why do some children handle the daily tasks and expectations of school with little to no anxiety, while others struggle to make it through the day? The answer is complicated. Dr. Elaine Aron, a clinical psychologist, discusses that children are born with a predisposition to sensitivity: highly emotional, fearful, sensitive to sensory, chaos, and stress. This sensitivity lasts a lifetime. Highly sensitive children who learn to manage their sensitivities are able to cope in situations that are difficult. However, sensitive children who have not been taught to handle discomfort and uncertainty struggle in life[5].

Few people have been educated on what anxiety really is. Before you can help a child (or yourself) you need to understand that anxiety is real and how it works in the body. Your brain has a small almond shaped "tool" called the amygdala, which is there to sense danger. It is located deep in the emotional section of your brain (the limbic system). Once the danger is encountered, the amygdala fires off the "fight or flight" response as a way to keep you safe and alive. It fires without any thought on your part, which is great in a real crisis. The amygdala is unable to differentiate between real and perceived danger, therefore, signally at any fear, anxiety, or danger. Of course, you want your amygdala firing off when a bear begins chasing you in the woods or when you need a boost of adrenaline when running in an important track event. However, it becomes a problem when it fires for each and every worrisome thought that enters the brain.

When the amygdala is fired, the prefrontal cortex of the brain, where rational thought and emotional regulation take place, shuts down and your body responds with fight or flight, or survival mode. A child experiencing anxiety at a level that triggers the amygdala is

---

[5] https://hsperson.com

truly unable to think rationally at the moment, making an instinctual move to either "fight" or "flight". The "fight" response looks like arguing, pushing materials or people out of their way, refusal, or defiance as a way to avoid whatever is causing the anxiety. The "flight" response is leaving the situation such as walking/running away from the anxiety-inducing event, seeking a safer place.

The problem with anxiety is that it quickly becomes habitual, making you feel ill-equipped to deal with the problem or situation. No child enjoys the feeling of anxiety, so they begin to avoid any situation in which they think that they may become anxious. This leads to avoidance, which strengthens anxiety and weakens the child's confidence in themselves, spiraling to an unhealthy situation. It is necessary to equip children with the idea that by facing anxiety, they can create new habits in the amygdala.

Here is an example of test anxiety. The child studies for the test. When given the test, their mind goes blank, leaving them anxious and feeling stupid. They do not score well on this test, telling themselves they will study harder next time. The next test rolls around. They are anxious about the upcoming test but study hard. The test arrives and they blank again, unable to complete the test. At this point, they believe that every time they have to take a test, they will panic. They have trained their amygdala that taking tests is a threat and should be feared. Therefore, they stop studying and begin avoiding test days either with sickness, behavior problems, or refusal.

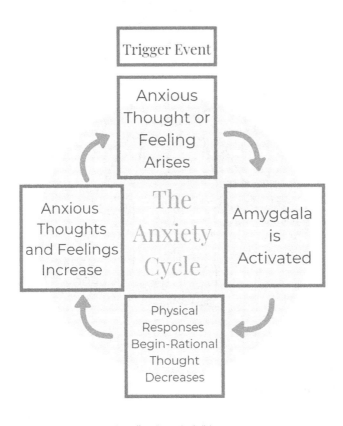

As anxiety creeps in, it creates physical sensations such as a racing heart, shallow breathing, sweatiness, shaky, dizziness, upset stomach, vomiting, diarrhea...the list goes on. These are real feelings that children are experiencing. Imagine how embarrassed a child feels to experience this while at school.

Physical Reactions To Anxiety

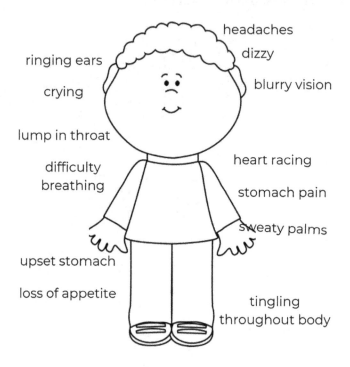

ringing ears

crying

headaches

dizzy

blurry vision

lump in throat

difficulty
breathing

heart racing

stomach pain

sweaty palms

upset stomach

loss of appetite

tingling
throughout body

https://goodbyeanxietyhellojoy.com

These awful feelings contribute to the need to avoid. Avoiding does not trigger anxiety, therefore, protecting the child from these unpleasant feelings. In addition to avoiding, anxious children rely on educators and parents for reassurance. The safety behaviors of avoidance and reassurance employed by anxious children create harmful long term effects. Avoidance trains the brain that events and activities are to be feared, causing more intense fear each time the avoidance occurs. This then leads to avoidance spreading into other situations and events in a child's life. Avoidance and reassurance impede children from learning how to problem solve, gain self-confidence, become independent, and form social connections.

Educators and parents have the best intentions when they support a child in avoiding or reassuring anxiety. Each of these safety behaviors provides immediate relief to the child, can happen quickly, and does not receive pushback from the child. However, educators and parents must step back and identify what, if any, safety behaviors are being used to enable an anxious child. It is easy to offer reassurance because you want to help the child find relief but remember the big picture...helping the child to learn to manage their anxiety in order to live their best life. Anxiety management is a skill that must be taught and practiced. Keep in mind that safety and avoidance will continue until a plan is implemented and a child learns the necessary skills. Even then, reassurance and avoidance are tapered off gradually.

Cycle of Avoidance and Reassurance with Anxiety

(Perceived) Scary Situation, Thought, or Feeling

Increased anxiety and avoidance

Response is to avoid or seek reassurance

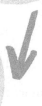

Reinforcement of negative response

https://goodbyeanxietyhellojoy.com

Exercise 4: What safety behaviors are you "accidentally" supporting in anxious children? Think deeply here to uncover any well-intentioned actions that you have taken that actually support the anxiety. Use exercise 4 to reference examples and brainstorm your safety behavior support.

Exercise 4
Do You Enable Safety Behaviors?
(Reassurance and Avoidance)

Child's Anxiety	Safety Behavior
Social anxiety transistioning in the hallway	Allow the child to leave 5 minutes early to avoid crowd
Child is afraid of spiders in any context	Allow child to leave the room when spiders are featured in a text

https://goodbyeanxietyhellojoy.com

Overcoming Anxiety

With a foundational understanding of anxiety and a consistent plan to manage it, children, with the support of parents and educators, can learn to manage their anxiety. Anxiety management focuses on learning skills to retrain the amygdala to fire only when real danger is encountered, rather than perceived danger. This skill is learned through practice. The skills are acquired slowly and with great patience. Forward progress takes place as skills are acquired. You, as an educator, hold the key to a child's success in overcoming intense anxiety and managing anxiety while at school. **Decreasing anxiety, through retraining the amygdala and engaging the prefrontal cortex, cannot be done through language. Children can not simply be told to do these steps and to think about the right things to do. They must actually DO THEM.** Their mindset must be of one that says, "Bring on the challenge, anxiety. I have got this!" These movements into anxiety are small baby steps, where educators and parents are figuratively or literally holding the child's hand as they step into the fear. The only way for a child to overcome anxiety at school (and at home) is through behaviors/experiences that create new, positive, memories for the brain.

Life is full of uncertainty and discomfort which is what anxious children need to learn to tolerate. **Without the tools and support in place, a child cannot be pushed into uncertain and uncomfortable situations.** The goal of creating a plan for a child's anxiety is not to eliminate the anxiety, but to teach and provide the skills needed to manage the anxiety. With educators and parents, and preferably the guidance of a trained therapist, anxious children gain the skills needed to cope with life's uncertainties. They learn to move into challenges rather than to avoid them. These scenarios, in the beginning, will heighten anxiety within the child, but since the child has been taught skills to cope with and manage anxiety, she is more capable of conquering the fear. With a child's newly acquired understanding that anxiety is manageable, he will strive to meet the goal of returning to typical activities that were once avoided due to anxiety. Educators and parents, children need you to guide and support them through these challenges as they grow and learn. You have the incredible opportunity to enthusiastically and skillfully change the course of a child's life through creating a consistent plan and using positive language. Like most good things in life, it takes time and patience. Please, do not give up on the anxious child. They need you. Every child deserves to come to school feeling safe, enjoying friends, and learning new ideas. A child with anxiety cannot do this without your unwavering, committed support.

You may be thinking...isn't this a parent issue? Yes, of course, it is. You definitely want the parents to understand what is happening in the classroom. Most children with severe anxiety will be showing signs at home as well. The best case scenario is that all adults work as a team, having the parents, educators, and hopefully a therapist, all on the same page. You should all be using the same language, routines, thought processes, encouragement, etc. The plan later in the book is a guide you can all use. However, not all families can afford therapy, nor do some have the time or ability to understand how to treat anxiety, so it may be on the school to help a child. That is ok. This guide will be very beneficial for you. Lastly, not all parents will support your view of what is seen in the classroom While this is not ideal, you can still make an incredible impact on a child while at school, which will carry over into their home life.

CHAPTER 2

Anxiety in the Classroom

Now that you have an understanding of anxiety and the important role that you play in a child's successful anxiety management, let's look at some examples an educator may see in the classroom. Very seldom will a child say, "I am anxious." It is up to you to recognize anxious behaviors and create a plan that addresses the anxiety in order to change unwanted and unpleasant behaviors. The anxiety felt by a child may be directly tied to school or it could be brought from home. Either way, if it is affecting the child while at school, you need to be there to help. Remember, no matter how frustrating it may be to teach a child with anxiety, that child hates the way that they feel and they want to feel better.

Common Types of Anxiety Seen at School

Separation Anxiety

Children are worried about being separated from caregivers, having a hard time at school drop-offs and throughout the day. A child who has a close bond with a teacher while at school may show signs of separation anxiety when leaving the teacher to transition to another place within the school. Children with this anxiety fear their safety when away from their caregiver or the safety of their loved ones when separated.

Social Anxiety

Children are excessively self-conscious, making it difficult for them to participate in class and socialize with peers. Any type of attention, group work, or crowds can cause intense anxiety in a child who fears being ridiculed, singled out, or embarrassed.

Selective Mutism

Children have a hard time speaking in some settings, like at school around the teacher. These children may talk when surrounded by close friends and family, but not in situations where they do not feel a strong bond.

Generalized Anxiety Disorder

Children worry about a wide variety of everyday things. This is often the term used for children who worry about many different things frequently.

Obsessive-Compulsive Disorder

Children's minds are filled with unwanted and stressful thoughts. Kids with OCD try to alleviate their anxiety by performing compulsive rituals. OCD can show itself in a wide variety of ways.

Specific Phobias

Children have an excessive and irrational fear of particular things, like dogs, storms, germs, or bugs.

Exercise 5: Use this checklist to mark any anxieties you are seeing in a child or children. Add notes to remind you of the behaviors that make you believe this type of anxiety may be present. Use exercise 5 to record your thoughts.

Exercise 5
Common Anxieties Seen at School

Check all that apply, add notes /thoughts of what you notice at school

☐ Separation Anxiety

☐ Social Anxiety

☐ Selective Mutism

☐ Generalized Anxiety Disorder

☐ Obsessive Compulsive Disorder

☐ Specific Phobias

☐ Other

https://goodbyeanxietyhellojoy.com

Comorbid Disorders with Anxiety

Anxiety can also be tied to the following disorders. Once again, it is not your job to diagnose these disorders, but it is important that you are aware of what children may be dealing with in your classroom. The information and strategies described throughout this book, while directed at anxiety, can benefit children with comorbid disorders as well (meaning disorders that are often seen along with anxiety).

Attention Deficit Hyperactivity Disorder (ADHD)

ADHD is one of the most common conditions for children in America, impacting focus, self-control, and other skills needed for daily life. In regards to schooling, it affects a child's ability to stay on task, organize their thoughts, control their emotions, access skills previously taught, flexible thinking, and self-regulation. Due to these issues, many children with ADHD also struggle with anxiety. They realize that they are unprepared for class, do not know the material being tested, call out when asked to be quiet, and so on. All of these behaviors and thoughts create self-doubt and anxiety in children with ADHD. While it is difficult to pinpoint if a child has anxiety, ADHD, or both since the behaviors are similar, the reality is that the information provided below will help a child with anxiety and ADHD be more successful in school. As a side note, it is important for parents to get a correct diagnosis if they plan to treat with medication, as stimulant medications often used for ADHD may heighten anxiety if it is present as well. In that case, non-stimulant medication can be used to help ADHD while not increasing anxiety.

Learning Disabilities

Children with any variety of learning disabilities face the greatest challenge, as their biggest fear is appearing "dumb" among their peers. With the increased pressure academically, these children continue to face immense anxiety as they work tirelessly to learn and master material that may simply be out of their capabilities. Dyslexia is the most common learning disability, which impacts reading and spelling. It has no impact on a child's general intelligence, but it makes learning basic skills incredibly challenging. Children with learning disabilities fear being called on to read, being embarrassed by their weak math or spelling skills, frustrations with the fact that they are misunderstood, or the pressure to perform timed tests. It is vitally important that children with learning disabilities be properly diagnosed and be taught using a systematic, research-based program specifically designed for their specific needs.

Autism Spectrum Disorders (ASD)

Nearly all children with autism will receive another diagnosis at some point. The most common comorbid diagnosis with autism is anxiety, affecting 40% of those with ASD. Even without an official diagnosis, anxiety is an important factor in the everyday lives of many children and teens with ASD. While it is hard to separate the anxiety from the traits of autism, it is possible to help children with autism manage parts of their anxiety while at school. For many children with ASD, anxiety is a result of their differences in how they relate to others, process information, and preference for a rigid schedule.

Trauma

Sadly, children in classrooms all around the world may be suffering from trauma, either from past experiences or current situations. Trauma can affect a child in many ways, often leading to a pattern of fearing their own self-worth, decisions, value, and future. They may shut down emotionally, being unable to use any type of coping strategy to handle a difficult situation. Depending on the trauma suffered, school can trigger anxiety based on the people in the child's life, news stories, peers, or activities taking place in the classroom.

Home Life

There is any number of events that can be taking place in a child's life that may cause anxiety at school. Children dealing with a parent's divorce, death of a loved one, violence in the home, lack of resources due to economic issues, illnesses within the family, and so on. Any of these events can cause a child to show signs of anxiety while at school. While this anxiety may not be at a level that leads to a diagnosis, and may improve as the situation at home improves, it is no less important that the child's anxiety be an important focus during the school day with the intention of helping that child work through the anxiety with little to no lasting effects.

Exercise 6: Use this checklist to mark any Comorbid Disorders that you are aware of in a child that may have anxiety. Record notes on what you see in that child as it relates to anxiety. Use exercise 6 to record your thoughts.

Exercise 6

Comorbid Disorders with Anxiety

Check all that apply, add notes /thoughts of what you notice at school

▢ ADHD

▢ Leaning Disability

▢ Autism Spectrum Disorder

▢ Trauma

▢ Home Life

▢ Other

Common Behaviors Tied to Anxiety

Anxiety is often disguised as something else, commonly ADHD or oppositional defiant disorder (ODD). While a child is battling anxiety, their rational thoughts escape, leaving them with only the tools needed to fight the anxiety that presents itself at the "fight or flight" level. This can lead to a lack of focus, fidgeting, a need to move, inability to listen to directions, crying, or repetitive actions. In more severe cases, a child feels such a need to flee the anxiety, that they use whatever means necessary to escape, possibly leaving a classroom or building. They are aware that the rules of school dictate that they stay in the classroom until permission is granted, but the anxiety is so strong that the rules are unable to be followed. At that moment, facing a consequence is a better option than continuing to feel the presence of anxiety. Many educators and parents see this as defiant behavior, as the child is defying expectations, but it is merely a loud cry for help.

Anxiety is never a cause for poor behavior and a child with anxiety should know that poor behavior is never acceptable. The expectation should always be that anxious or not, actions should be school appropriate. Here is the challenge, poor behaviors will happen with anxiety until the child is given the skills needed to handle the anxiety properly, and time is given to master the new skills. Simply consequencing the inappropriate behavior choice in the hopes that the negative consequence will lead to better choices will not happen with anxiety. An anxious child is desperate to avoid the anxiety and therefore, without skills or support, will do the only thing they know how to do, which is to avoid. As an educator or a parent, this is really frustrating and weakens your patience. This is why you need to create a plan that can be followed by everyone involved. It takes away the guesswork and spontaneity that arise with anxiety. A consistent plan creates structure and calmness, allowing the anxious child to learn the skills needed to handle the discomfort and uncertainty of life.

Needy and Dependent

Anxious children seem to only see the negative in life. As mentioned, anxiety leads to self-confidence issues and avoidance of events in life. With these two issues weighing down on a child, they begin to see the world in a negative light. Suddenly, everyone is mean, they have no friends, all of their clothes are ugly, they are stupid, and so much more. This all makes sense since anxiety is overtaking their thoughts, making it hard to focus on happiness and good in the world. They catastrophize their life and only see things as black and white.

Similarly, anxiety strips children of their confidence and independence. They appear very needy and insecure. To compensate they are constantly seeking validation, often asking for help to complete a task (which they are capable of doing themselves). Also, having lost their confidence, they take things personally and overreact to comments about their appearance, school work, performances, abilities, etc. You will often hear, "Are you mad at me?", "Do you like me?", or "It's all my fault". They are asking this, needing to hear that they are cared for and supported.

Lack of focus- Inattentive

Children who are anxious often come across as inattentive or unfocused. Many anxious children will be diagnosed with ADHD before being diagnosed with anxiety. This is not to say that ADHD is not present, but it may not be the root cause. A child feeling anxious will become fidgety and unfocused as they attempt to find ways to handle their anxiety. Anxiety can cause a physical need to move, therefore, you may notice their legs bouncing, hands wringing, or their entire body fidgeting. Additionally, an anxious child may be so focused on their thoughts and not the activities or lessons happening around them. They are easily distracted by what is going on. Anxious children may appear to zone out, fall behind academically, or be unable to sit still.

Attendance Issues

Children with anxiety issues will often miss many days of school or come to school late. They have physical symptoms caused by anxiety, which lead those around them to believe they are ill. These physical symptoms may be tied to anxiety over separating from their parents, worries about an upcoming test, or issues within their peer group. For children with school refusal, the parent is unable to get their child out of the house and into school, therefore missing excessive days of school.

For children who do come to school anxious, they spend a large amount of time out of the classroom, either in the guidance office, with the nurse, or in another calm space. While there are times that anxious children may need a break, time spent outside of the classroom can actually increase their anxiety as they fall behind academically.

Disruptive, Anger

Anxious children are in a constant state of fight or flight due to their mind's perceived threat of danger. This state leads to an overly active nervous system leaving them exhausted and unable to regulate their emotions properly. Often, they will react with intense anger and frustration over minor situations that arise. They are simply so worn out from battling the perceived threat, that they cannot handle anything else. Think of an overtired toddler who cries and throws tantrums for no reason, the same concept applies here- exhaustion!

Similarly, anxiety brings such an intense fear to children that they are willing to do almost anything to avoid the event or activity that causes the anxious feeling. This includes being defiant and misbehaving. The fear of "getting in trouble" or "facing punishment or consequence" is less feared than doing the "right thing" because the "right thing" leads to the anxious feeling. Children know that the decision to misbehave or defy is wrong, but the need to avoid the anxiety is stronger. Once the poor behavior decision is made, they often feel immense guilt. An anxious child may run away, hide, refuse to do school work, avoid going to school or an activity, all because of the intense fear of what is waiting for them.

Trouble Answering Questions or Completing Work

For children with anxiety centered around perfectionism, mistake making, or embarrassment, answering questions when called upon or completing an assignment can trigger their anxiety. The result is that they refuse to answer the questions being asked and avoid the work that was assigned. This may also be seen in their lack of completing homework assignments.

Refusal, Defiance, Need for Control

Anxiety floods the mind with scary and overwhelming thoughts. It makes children feel helpless. In order to overcome the anxious thoughts and the feeling of helplessness, they begin to control whatever they can. It helps them feel a bit more control given the strength of the anxiety. They will do all they can to control a situation by overplanning for events, refusing to compromise, and being overly "bossy" in their relationships with family and friends.

A child with anxiety will fight to avoid any anxiety-inducing event such as writing, test taking, going into the cafeteria, entering a classroom where someone was recently ill, attending an assembly, and so on. While the child is aware that refusing or defying the set expectations at school is not appropriate, without anxiety management skills, to them, the only option for relief is to avoid the task.

Power struggles often happen when refusal, defiance, and need for control arise, as the educator or parent sees this as manipulation and misbehavior. While there is truth to that, there is no amount of negotiating, bribery, or compromise that will allow the adult to have their agenda followed when anxiety is the reason for the choices made by the child.

Frequent Complaints of Physical Symptoms and Requests to Visit the Nurse

With the overuse of the nervous system (fight or flight), physical symptoms are real. Anxious children often complain about headaches, stomachaches, nausea, or feeling overly tired. You will probably notice a pattern of when these complaints happen. It may happen each morning before school, when a child is getting ready for their sporting event, before bed at night, or when you go to a store or restaurant. While these physical complaints are tied to anxiety rather than another medical issue, they are real feelings to the child. More severe anxiety may result in complaints of dizziness, chest pain, or trouble breathing. These could be signs of a panic attack. When a child frequently visits the nurse, the nurse needs to be part of the plan in order to keep the consistency of working towards anxiety management rather than using the nurse as an avoidance mechanism.

Avoiding Peers

Children who struggle with social anxiety and phobias may find it hard to be around peers due to their fear of embarrassment or germs. These children desperately want to be a part of the class and want to create friendships but they find themselves often working, playing, and sitting alone. When assigned group work, they often refuse to be a part of the group, choosing to work alone. On the playground and in the cafeteria you will often see these children separate from their peers.

Continually Questioning or "What Ifs"

Children with anxiety ask questions excessively in order to prepare and plan for what may be coming. They are trying to make sense of a situation and gain a sense of control. The same questions may be asked repeatedly to ensure that they are fully prepared for the event. Excessive questioning may also be tied to the need for reassurance that they are safe, healthy, or taken care of. The word "excessive" is key here...children by nature are curious and will often ask questions. In addition to questions about concrete situations, a child may ask "What ifs?" excessively. You may begin to notice that these questions are centered around a particular situation such as weather, school pick up, or an illness. These "What ifs?" are being asked to help the child gain an understanding of an anxiety-inducing situation or event they are dealing with internally.

It is important to note that these behaviors are not a direct indicator of anxiety, but they are frequently tied to anxiety. Often a child may exhibit these behaviors at a specific time of day or during a certain activity. In this case, a child may not have an anxiety disorder, but can still be dealing with anxiety. There is no need to label a child as "anxious" when you notice these behaviors. The idea is to recognize that anxiety may be playing a role, formulate a plan for helping the child work through the discomfort in order to succeed academically, emotionally, physically.

One very difficult aspect of behavior and anxiety is that educators often do not see the correlation between the two due to the uniqueness of anxiety. A child may act "typical" with no signs of anxiety during certain situations, but then act out with inappropriate behaviors in another situation. On that same note, for some children, anxiety may be present one day in a specific situation, and not there the next day. This makes it very challenging to understand and anticipate anxiety. Depending on the intensity and severity of the anxiety, it may not always be present. This should not diminish the importance of dealing with it properly when it is present in the child.

Defiance and Misbehavior refusal to comply to avoid anxiety inducing situation	Inattention lack of focus, slipping grades, fidgeting, easily distracted	Need for Control over planning, controlling situations, unwilling to compromise	Physical Symptoms stomachaches, headaches, overly tired

10
Not So Obvious Signs of Anxiety in Children

Seeking Validation feelings of neediness and insecurity

Good Bye Anxiety, Hello Joy

Anger and Frustration constantly in a state of perceived danger

Negative Nelly sees the negative in all situations, exaggerates the negative, unable to see positive	Sleep Issues trouble falling sleep, waking often, not wanting to sleep alone	Avoidance not participating in events, school activities, sports, family outings	Excessive Question Asking seeking reassurance and formulating a plan

Exercise 7: Write down some behaviors that you have observed previously or are observing currently. Note what the behavior looks like, when it occurs, and how it had been/or is being handled. Use exercise 7 to record your observations.

Exercise 7

Behaviors Observed in Children at School
(This is not specific to a child...just general behaviors
seen at school)

Behaviors Observed- what does it look like	When are these behaviors occurring?	How are these behaviors currently handled?
Refusal to complete work, head down, arguing	During independent math work	Missed choice time, email sent home, lower grades

https://goodbyeanxietyhellojoy.com

Exercise 8: Now that you have completed chapters 1 and 2, gaining an understanding of anxiety, how have your thoughts and ideas surrounding anxiety changed? Have your opinions on the role of a teacher, in regards to supporting anxious children, changed? Use exercise 10 to record your beliefs about anxiety after reading these chapters.

Exercise 8 focuses on understanding your thoughts about anxiety AFTER reading these chapters.

New ideas and thoughts I have about anxiety now...	How does this information change my perspective about anxiety?

Anxiety

I believe my role in supporting a child with anxiety is...	Biggest ah-ha moment while reading this was...

https://goodbyeanxietyhellojoy.com

CHAPTER 3

An Educator's Role in Supporting a Child with Anxiety

Your job as an educator is to create a classroom environment where all children can succeed. The ideas in this chapter benefit the mental health of all children in the class, as they reduce stress and anxiety while improving much-needed personal skills. For children who are anxious, you will want to bump this up when talking with them personally, delving a bit deeper to really drive the point home. In order to create a classroom full of confident, independent learners, with or without anxiety, you will focus on creating an environment where the mental health needs of children are prioritized.

Create Secure Student-Educator Relationships

Hopefully, you know that the student-educator relationship is the single most important factor for a child's success in school. From the first meeting between an educator and a child, the educator must build a relationship where the educator is sensitive and responsive to a child's needs. Children with anxiety may be hesitant about creating this relationship. The educator needs increased patience and creative ways to build the bond. As a secure bond forms between the two, a child begins to trust and respect their teacher. This feeling of safety greatly reduces feelings of anxiety.

A bond is built through verbal language, body language, facial expression, and tone, and the educator showing that he or she understands and accepts a child for who they are. A child with anxiety needs to know that the teacher "gets" them and is there to help them throughout the school day.

Here are some ways that educators can strengthen their relationships with all children:

- Be authentic. Let children see your mistakes and weaknesses while also being proud of your strengths.
- Use humor in the classroom as often as possible. It creates a fun, relaxing environment and relieves stress.
- Spend time getting to know children as individuals, rather than a "student" or a number.
- Listen attentively and make time for personal relationships to develop throughout the day.
- Never give up on a child no matter how challenging the relationship feels.

Configure the Classroom for Success

Overhead Lighting

Dimming overhead lighting and adding lamps can improve the overall mood of children. Too much bright light is incredibly stimulating for their brains. This can lead to over-stimulation by the end of the day. Their bodies need light, but it should be natural and subtle. When possible, remove curtains from windows, allowing natural light to fill the classroom. Supplement with lamps throughout the room. If lamps are not an option, you can purchase light cover filters through school supply catalogs. The overall feeling of the classroom will become calm with just this one change.

Essential Oil Diffuser

Purchase an essential oil diffuser, allowing you to diffuse calming oils such as lavender, Valor, or peppermint throughout the day. Essential oils are shown to calm anxieties, increase focus and wakefulness, and even help fight germs. Children enjoy the scent that fills the classroom, making it an inviting place to be. As you learn more about oils, you will be able to diffuse different oils depending on your schedule for the day...are you testing, is there a lot of sicknesses, has the weather been keeping children inside for recess? No matter what the situation, there is an oil for it!

Weighted Lap Pads

Weighted lap pads and sensory objects should be available in all classrooms for children to use when needed. These weighted pads are similar to weighted blankets but smaller in size. They apply deep touch pressure to a child when placed on their lap in a seated position. This deep pressure has been shown to improve attention, calm anxieties and help children relax. There are a variety of pads on the market from small rectangular blankets to cute weighted stuffed animals. These are not to be used all day, just when a child needs support in regulating their bodies.

Fidgets

Fidgets are useful for a variety of reasons and range from small cubes to sequenced textured throw pillows. They allow children who are struggling with anxiety or attention issues to self-soothe through the repetitive motion and/or tactile feeling, often removing distractions, either physical or mental. Without the distractions, anxiety can be better managed and attention can return to the task as planned. Another type of fidget would be to use stretchy resistance bands tied around the legs of a stable chair. The band allows movement for a child who "plays " with it using his or her feet. Fidgets should not be used as a toy, which would lead to distracting behaviors.

Music

With the accessibility of technology in classrooms, music can be used either individually or throughout the entire classroom. Slow music can help lower anxieties and hyperactivity, and increase focus. Children who have access to iPads or Chromebooks can utilize music as needed with earphones. Classroom teachers can play music for the entire class through speakers, Smartboards, or Apple TV systems. Some Youtube channels offer calming music with serene scenery for those who may benefit from the visual effects as well. The Calm App also offers a free subscription for teachers to use in their classrooms.

Flexible Seating

Flexible seating is a newer concept that allows a variety of seating options and locations throughout the classroom for children. Allowing children to choose their own seat gives them ownership over their space as well as the ability to select a seat or location that physically feels good. Classrooms can have standard chairs, rocking chairs, wobbly stools, bean bag chairs, or even small carpet squares. Like fidgets, rocking chairs and wobbly stools allow children the movement that is needed in order for them to learn. Similarly, creating a calm space in the classroom with rugs or carpet squares give children a safe place to sit when dealing with overwhelming feelings.

Movement Breaks

Studies show that movement improves brain function and reduces anxiety. Adding structured movement breaks into the school day allow opportunities for children to stretch, wiggle, and relax their mind. You can buy kid-friendly yoga cards to create a short routine after recess, introduce children to the crab walk or wall push-ups after a long assignment, or subscribe to a movement channel such as "Go Noodle" to use as needed. As with any activity, expectations should be clearly defined in order to keep the movement breaks productive for all children.

These simple classroom improvements will make the overall environment more enjoyable for everyone. Anxious children will benefit from the calmer atmosphere created by more natural light, uplifting oils, and relaxing music.

Normalize Anxiety

Anxiety, worries, and fears are seldom discussed as they are often seen as a sign of weakness. As children grow, they work hard to avoid being embarrassed by their peers. Although many children sleep with nightlights, are scared of storms, and fear the dark, seldom do they admit it. As an educator and parent, you have an opportunity to normalize fears and worries.

From the first day of school, mention moments of uncertainty and discomfort from your own life, how you felt, and how you got through those situations. For most of us, these feelings happen throughout the day, some more problematic and intense than others.

On the first day of school each year, I always told children that I was super excited to be their teacher and I loved the first day of school, but I admitted that I was very nervous. Each year the children's facial expressions registered their shock, that I, as a teacher, was scared for the first day of school. I described my excitement at meeting them but also the butterflies in my stomach because I wondered if the children would like me, what if I didn't remember their names, and what if I forgot our new schedule. I often read a story about the first day of school. (There is a list of literature to share with children at the end of this book.) By doing this, I was normalizing the fears and uncertainty that many other children also felt. It allowed children to express their concerns for the first day. Hearing stories from other kids helps everyone. This is not to say I created a negative, sad atmosphere, instead, it was relaxed as I created a classroom environment where feelings were shared and accepted.

This dialogue continued throughout the year. Your attitude and view of the problem are important. You must word them in a way that, while expressing anxiety, shows that you have the knowledge and confidence to create a plan and a mindset to work through whatever situation you are faced with. For a child with anxiety, it is important to have shared these honest, real-life stories with children throughout the year because you can access them when a child is struggling. When you see an anxious child, find out what is causing their worries (if they are able to articulate it), then remind them how you handled a similar situation in your life. This will help them normalize whatever it is they are feeling. Now, this may not completely defuse the anxiety, meaning, it may be intense enough that more tools are needed, but it continues to set the stage that we all deal with similar thoughts and feelings at times and come through without a problem.

By sharing stories of your own life, allowing children to share their stories, and providing literature on this topic, children learn that while life is full of opportunities for discomfort and uncertainty which create anxiety, these feelings are normal and can be solved. This leads to problem-solving which is needed for all children, but especially children who struggle with anxiety.

Exercise 9: Collect ideas of stories you can share with children highlighting times you were worried or uncomfortable. How did you handle these situations and move on? Record your thoughts on exercise 9.

Exercise 9
Personal Experiences of Uncertainty/Discomfort

Event	Outcome
Traffic back up on the way to work so I was late	I was worried about arriving to school after the children arrived. I called the school and explained the situation. The secretary promised someone would be in the classroom to greet children.

https://goodbyeanxietyhellojoy.com

Use Positive Language

Language and tone used in the classroom are important for every child. This does not mean that you are expected to be sugar sweet with how and what you say. The idea is that no matter what children express to you, your language and tone support your respect and understanding of the problem they are facing. Often, especially with younger children, they can be very upset over the smallest moment or detail. It is not your job to decide how important this really is or how affected or emotional they should be. It is all about perception. If a child perceives an event or situation as anxious or uncomfortable, while you have no idea how that could be so, it is real to them.

Keep in mind that when a child is anxious, their rational brain is not functioning properly. Their actions and behaviors are a result of the fight or flight response. In these cases, asking a child "why" he or she did what they did will not provide a clear answer. Most of the time, they are not able to articulate why they made the decision. Older children may be able to identify that the choice they made was a result of anxiety, but this is not common. When you ask a child this question, expecting an answer, you frustrate the child even more, as they are already upset with the anxiety and what it has lead to. For example, a child who acts up in class, yelling out silly phrases and clowning around while she is supposed to be working, will not tell you that those actions and behaviors were a response to the anxiety felt when she did not know how to correctly finish the assignment.

The language and attitude in which you respond set the tone for how a situation or event will move forward from that moment. All children, but especially those who are already anxious about any variety of topics, will pick up on the way in which you choose to approach a topic.

It is very important to avoid generalized and catastrophic statements such as, "you will never get into college without taking these classes", "you must pass this test to move to the next grade", "this is the most important assignment you will ever have", etc. Too many children (including teens) take these statements literally and as fact. For a child already stressed, these statements add an incredible amount of pressure.

The following two phrases should be wiped out of your vocabulary. They come easily off the tongue, and the intention behind them may be positive, but they never lead to success.

"Calm down."

Simply asking a child to "calm down" is insulting. It implies that she can turn off the anxiety and return to the task at hand. No child would choose to feel anxious and out of control...she is trying to "calm down" but is past the rational stage that would allow her the ability to simply calm down. If you remember this each and every time you interact with an anxious child, you are already more helpful than most people! No matter how frustrated you become, think about how awful the child feels having to experience their anxiety. Empathy and understanding is a must for anything you learn from this point forward to be effective.

"You are fine."

No, they are not fine. They are feeling scared and out of control. As an adult, you know "they are fine", meaning that their current reaction is caused by anxiety rather than some true life-threatening situation, but they are not "fine". They are suffering.

As you wipe out the above phrases and replace them with the following, a more productive resolution will happen. These phrases show you care and understand what the child is going through at that moment.

- "What do you need?"
- "You are safe."
- "I care about you."
- "I know this feels bad, but it will pass."
- "You are doing really well at _____."

"What do you need?"

Asking a child what he needs empowers him to ask for anything that will assist in working through the anxiety. Each child is different and has different tools and techniques for working through an anxious moment. It is important to remember that each anxiety attack may also call for different tools to assist.

"You are safe."

Reminding children that their feelings are real but that they are not in any danger assures them that they are safe. Remind them that you are there to take care of them and keep them safe. Equally important is to remind them that they are safe because they have the skills to take care of themselves during these difficult thoughts and feelings. They may not be able to independently get through these anxious moments, but continue to empower them to believe in themselves by reminding them of their own ability to feel safe.

"I care about you."

Simply reminding a child that you care about him when he is at his worst can lessen the burden being felt. Often children with anxiety lack confidence in themselves and feel guilty about how their anxiety is affecting those around them. They need to be reminded that you care for them all of the time, even when challenges arise.

"I know this feels bad now, but it will pass."

This statement shows the child that you acknowledge how she is feeling rather than dismissing it. It also reminds her that the anxious feeling will not go on forever. Once again, continue to empower the child that by using their skills to cope with anxiety they will move through the unpleasant thoughts and feelings.

"You are doing really well at _____."

For example, "you are doing a great job at slowing your breathing" or "going for a walk was a great idea." The positive compliments show that you see the hard work the child is putting into managing their anxiety. This helps build their confidence in themselves to handle the anxiety when it arises.

Exercise 10: Think of examples of negative language you may be using in the classroom. What can you use instead that is more positive? (Do not feel bad about the negative language. We all do it, even when we know better. The goal is to bring attention to your language and create the habit of using positive language frequently.) Use exercise 10 to collect your thoughts.

Examples of Negative Language I Use

> • You will be fine. Your stomach always hurts when we do math. Go sit down and keep working hard.

Examples of Positive Language I Can Use

> • I am sorry your stomach hurts. It seems like you are worried about math again. What can I do to help you?

https://goodbyeanxietyhellojoy.com

Teach Problem Solving Skills and Emotional Intelligence

The goal is to teach children to become creative, independent thinkers with a strong sense of emotional intelligence in order to solve their own problems. Just as you model working through the everyday uncertainties and discomforts in your life, you should also model your thought process for problem-solving when applicable.

There are two parts to this: Solving the problem and strengthening emotional intelligence which is explained in more detail below.

All children face challenges, problems, and discomfort at some point each day. It may be a challenging reading passage, difficulty opening the packaging of their snack, forgetting their locker combination, or feeling angry at a friend. You must teach children how to solve these problems when they arise since you are unable to solve every problem for them. It takes time, practice, and maturity to become independent problem solvers. However, for children with anxiety, their ability to solve problems is very weak. Rather than putting their energy into solving the problem, they may invest their time in avoiding the issue. As anxious children become problem solvers, it tends to lower their anxiety in many situations which leads to increased independence and confidence.

Solving the problem: These steps should be taught to all children and placed in a visible location in the classroom (or home) as a reminder. For many anxious children, these steps can be used during structured breaks (which will be part of the plan you create) to work through the anxiety caused by the problem.

1. Identify the problem- Verbalize or write down the problem. For example: "I forgot my homework at home and it is due today. Now I will get in trouble."

2. List at least 4 solutions to the problem- These do not have to be feasible solutions, just any ideas that come to mind. For example: "I could call my mom. I could walk home and get it. I could talk to the teacher and see if I can turn it in tomorrow. I could ask for another copy and do it at recess."

3. Talk through the pros and cons of each of the ideas- Listen to the child share their thoughts and then add your own only if something needs clarifying or expounded upon. For example: "My mom is at work so she probably will not be able to leave work and bring it to me. I live too far away to walk home. The teacher will like that I am honest and will probably let me turn it in late although I may lose a few points. I could do it at recess but I really want to play with my friends."

4. Pick the best solution- This can be tricky because kids with anxiety may not want to pick any of the solutions, as they may see something "wrong" with every idea. In this case, help guide them towards the best solution to their problem. For example: "I guess turning it in tomorrow is the best idea here but I am not happy that I may lose a few points for being late."

5. Revisit the problem/solution once the action is completed to decide if the solution was successful. If not, discuss what can be done in the future in similar situations.

This simple outline for problem-solving can be used for nearly every situation a child encounters. Over time and through practice, the majority of the minor problems with be solved without the needed steps above. However, for bigger problems, helping a child solve them rather than solving it for them leads to less anxiety and greater confidence and independence. The image below shows one of the bonus worksheets available as a downloadable PDF.

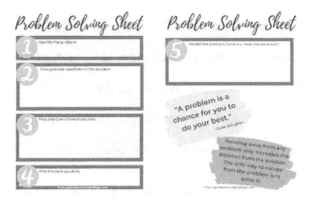

Emotional intelligence refers to the understanding, awareness, and ability to express emotions. Children under 10 use very few emotions to express their thoughts and feelings. As they grow and mature, they have the ability to use and express a more varied approach to emotions. Again, anxious children struggle to understand and manage their emotions in useful and appropriate ways.

Adults tend to create the idea that some emotions are good, while others are bad. It is important that children (and adults) understand that emotions are neither positive or negative. They are a critical part of who we are and how we feel. Many anxious children are so used to feeling "scared" that they label nearly every emotion in the same manner. It is important that they realize they may be feeling sad, hungry, tired, or angry rather than scared. The different emotions, when recognized, allow for different ways of dealing with their feelings. Being scared leads to fight or flight, but other emotions do not often trigger that same response.

Many children (and adults) stick to basic words to describe their emotions...sad, happy, mad. Yet, there are hundreds of words that can be used to describe what children are feeling, offering a more accurate take on what is happening inside their minds and bodies.

You can model the use of deep emotional vocabulary by making sure to share your emotions more clearly and accurately.

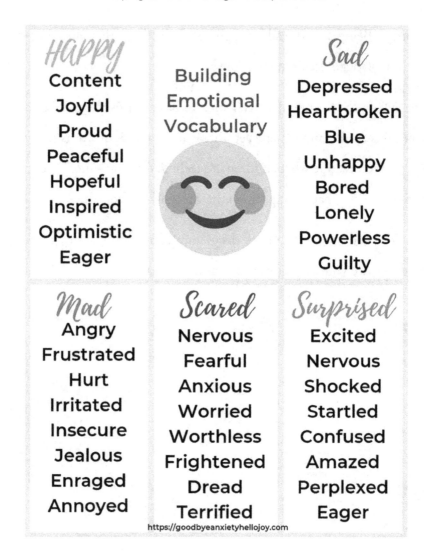

HAPPY
Content
Joyful
Proud
Peaceful
Hopeful
Inspired
Optimistic
Eager

Building Emotional Vocabulary

Sad
Depressed
Heartbroken
Blue
Unhappy
Bored
Lonely
Powerless
Guilty

Mad
Angry
Frustrated
Hurt
Irritated
Insecure
Jealous
Enraged
Annoyed

Scared
Nervous
Fearful
Anxious
Worried
Worthless
Frightened
Dread
Terrified

Surprised
Excited
Nervous
Shocked
Startled
Confused
Amazed
Perplexed
Eager

https://goodbyeanxietyhellojoy.com

Praise Effort Over Result

All children in your classroom have strengths and weaknesses. This is why it is so important to praise and celebrate effort over results. Too often, teachers praise the high grades on math tests with an extra recess or celebrate the memorization of math facts with an ice cream party. For the children who did not receive the expected grade or the proficient memorization of math facts, being left out is an awful feeling. The goal for any educator is to strive for mastery of the material by all children. However, the reality is that growth and effort are far more important than immediate mastery.

Anxious children work hard all day, every day and it is mentally and physically exhausting. More often than not, they just want to give up and avoid because, in the moment, it seems easier. It is vitally important that everyone around this child celebrate all of the efforts, no matter how small. Maybe an anxious child was not able to complete the test he attempted to take, but the effort for trying should be celebrated. Any time that you see a child doing parts of the plan, managing the anxiety in an appropriate manner, or working through an uncomfortable situation, praise their effort with specific praise. For example, "I saw you taking a few deep breaths before entering the hallways. I am really proud of you for accessing that skill and making it to your next class on time." We all know the value of praising individual effort for academic progress, the same is true for anxiety management.

All of the suggestions mentioned in this chapter focused on ways to create a classroom environment that improves the mental health and overall success for every child. For some children with anxiety, these improvements will be enough to overcome their mild anxieties. However, children with more intense anxiety, while benefiting greatly from these enhancements, will still need more individualized support. The next chapter focuses on creating a plan for these specific children.

CHAPTER 4

Creating Individual Plans for Children to Manage Anxiety at School

The last chapter focused on ways to create a classroom environment benefitting the mental health of all children, especially those with anxiety. This chapter focuses on the extra effort that needs to be taken to help children who are experiencing levels of anxiety at school impacting their academics, social skills, and emotional well being. Always keep in mind that anxiety will look different in each child and can even change day by day within the same child. The key is to focus closely on the fact that the child has anxiety and less on the behaviors and triggers. For example, a child with a fear of germs will be treated with a plan very similar to a child fearful of crowds. This is because anxiety is predictable and similar in nearly all cases. Anxiety creates physical and mental reactions that lead to avoidance. The goal is not necessarily to be comfortable with germs or crowds but to understand anxiety and have the skills to use whenever feelings of discomfort arise.

The plan that you create will give the child the ability to manage anxiety in nearly all situations once the necessary skills are taught. **Before children move into anxious situations, they must understand what is happening in their mind and body, their ability to manage anxiety, and the positive outcomes that result from their hard work.**

Due to the unique and varying anxieties that are seen in children, it would be impossible to create an exact plan that would be applicable to all children with anxiety. The information below is very precise, in the attempt to touch on every minute detail that needs to be considered for a child. Seldom will everything presented below need to be included in a plan for a child with anxiety. Most times, bits and pieces have been slapped together over the years either by parents, therapists, or the school, in an attempt to help the child be more successful and less anxious. In this case, your job is to use the information you have learned about anxiety in order to find the gaps in the previous plans that have been in place for this child. Once the gaps are found that have contributed to unsuccessful anxiety management, you will be able to create a solid plan. A previous plan can be anything, formal or informal, that has been designed or discussed as a way to help a child. From this point on, you want to create a formal plan, hopefully as an IEP or 504, that can be shared with every person on this child's team, and can be used as a tool for accountability that the child is receiving all resources necessary as she overcomes her anxiety in order to succeed at school.

The idea is always to create a plan that teaches the child to **understand and manage** their anxiety, not a plan that feeds the anxiety through reassurance and avoidance. As you know from classroom management education and experience, it always takes time and patience to create and implement a new plan because you must do a bit of trial and error and give it time to show its effectiveness. Be prepared for push back from the child in the beginning, but with a well thought out plan, authentic support within the school, and (hopefully) parental and therapeutic support outside of the school, a child will learn to manage their anxiety at school.

At all times while working with an anxious child, their mental health should be the focus, followed by social relationships, than academics. There is no reason to pressure a child with intense anxiety to focus on the lesson being taught or the work that needs to be completed while they are attempting to manage their anxiety in an appropriate way. This idea is very hard to accept for parents and educators but it is necessary for success. The goal should always be to attend classes, even when academic work is not being completed. This doesn't mean you shouldn't include the anxious child in the lessons or assign him the work, however, if a child is not responsive, do not push it. Classwork can be modified into smaller chunks, different presentation methods offered or allow extended time to complete the work. As the anxiety improves, so should the expectation to complete full assignments, on time, without modifications. Depending on a child's anxiety, the incomplete classwork can be sent home to finish or worked on with tutors outside of school. It could also be considered exempt. Remember, anxiety management is a process leading to long term success. The time put in now, will pay off later. The academics missed during this time seldom has long term negative effects. Similarly, for children on a modified school schedule from a public school, the district should provide home instruction where the child will work with a teacher outside of school hours for their academic lessons.

Social relationships are also more important than academics for children, especially those working through anxiety. Humans crave connection, meaning it is essential for positive mental health. As anxious children manage their anxiety successfully, they begin to reconnect with their peers finding themselves wanting to be around their friends and classmates. Having these positive connections continues to encourage them to be in class. As children spend more time in the classroom setting due to positive anxiety management, rather than avoiding, they are motivated to connect with others. This connection drives them to continue working hard to overcome their anxiety at school. Once a child is settled back into the routine of attending class, their anxiety is minimal, and they have reconnected with their peers, the academics can once again be expected like it would of any other child at their ability level.

Collecting Data

Now that you understand anxiety, are aware of common anxieties and comorbid disorders, behaviors that arise with anxiety, and the impact your classroom environment has on anxiety, it is time to learn how to create a successful plan for the child struggling with anxiety. You are encouraged to finish the entire book before beginning to create the plan, however, you do need to begin collecting data now (sheet provided) in order to best understand this particular child's anxiety and needs in order to put an individualized plan together. You should collect data for at least a week, longer if time allows. Once you have all the data, you will be able to meet with parents and other school personnel to share your knowledge and insight.

Exercise 11: Use the data collection sheet to gain a clear picture of an individual child's anxious behavior. Be as precise as possible when collecting data. (The data sheet shown here is intended for the educator or parent. There is a similar sheet for the child in the collection of bonus worksheets.)

Exercise 11
Individual Data Collection

Child:

Time Place	
Actions and/or behaviors witnessed	
What was occurring before the behaviors? What was coming after the behaviors occured?	
How were these behaviors handled?	

https://goodbyeanxietyhellojoy.com

In addition to collecting data on the child's anxious behaviors during school, it is important to have clear, up to date, information about the child's experience with anxiety up to this point. Before creating a plan for a child, you must have details from parents and outside therapists, when applicable, highlighting what the child already knows about how anxiety relates to them personally. Find out if the child sees a therapist, the language and concepts used during these sessions, and what the parent does at home to support their child's anxiety.

Creating the Team

First, educators, reach out to parents. (Parents if you are reading this with the intention of meeting with the school, then you will reach out to the school with the information that you have learned.) If parents have not notified you about anxiety, be sure to communicate what you are seeing in the classroom. Often, parents will be seeing similar things at home. They may or may not realize that it could be anxiety. The hope is that educators and parents agree to work together, and even better, have the child seen by a medical professional, either for diagnosis if needed, or therapy.

If parents are unwilling to work with you, you are still able to create a plan between you and the child to help him while at school.

Think about who within the school can be a part of this child's support team. It is necessary to have at least one additional person, besides the classroom teacher, who is available to the anxious child **whenever** she needs support outside of the classroom. Seldom are school staff members readily available in one location due to their various responsibilities to other children. Really think this through! A child with anxiety must feel confident that someone is available to support them when they need it most.

If you select a guidance counselor or nurse to be the specified staff member to support this child, what happens when the guidance counselor is meeting with another child or working in a classroom? What happens if the nurse's office is closed for lunch? These are important ideas to keep in mind when designating a staff member as the "on call" support staff for an anxious child.

It is highly unlikely, and unfair to everyone, that a classroom teacher is expected to help a child manage their anxiety within the classroom unless the child's anxiety is very minor and infrequent. Children who need an individual plan to be put in place as they learn the skills needed to manage their anxiety, deserve structured, focused attention. A classroom teacher, with a room full of children, cannot give the anxious child the time or attention that he deserves. This is why another staff member must be available for the anxious child whenever the anxiety strikes.

Keep in mind that the intense support an anxious child needs, in the beginning, will decrease as the child learns and understands how he is able to independently manage the anxiety. It is well worth it, in the long run, to put the necessary time and energy into supporting this child from the start as you will see long term successful anxiety management when a well thought out plan is implemented and followed with consistency and validity.

For children whose parents are already aware of the anxiety, it is important to meet to discuss what you are seeing in the classroom, what parents are seeing at home, and what is already being done to help this child manage anxiety. The most successful way to help a child is to have the parents, school, and therapist (when there is one) all working towards a common goal using the same language, ideas, and encouragement. If there is a current plan that needs revised, use this information to share what you know about anxiety and how you would like to help the child while at school.

It is important to keep in mind that the level of anxiety, the length of time in which anxiety has been creating bad habits, and the school's and parent's attitude and involvement toward anxiety are going to impact the plan moving forward. A child who may only become anxious during a test is going to be easier to work with and devise a plan for than a child suffering from generalized anxiety disorder or OCD.

Depending on the child, the school and parent support, and the experience with a therapist, a child may want to offer her ideas to the plan. It is important to include the child when it can be beneficial. As a note, many children do not want a plan to manage anxiety because it is very scary and difficult to work through the anxious thoughts and feelings. They would rather avoid, which will not be supported in this plan. If a child is resistant, do not include them in this part. They will have an important role later.

Teaching the Child to Understand Anxiety

Explain Anxiety and Its Effect on the Child

The first step in helping a child manage their anxiety effectively begins by providing the child with a concrete, detailed understanding of anxiety and how it relates to them. The way in which you educate a child will vary depending on the child's age, past experiences, and their attitude towards anxiety. That being said, even young children should be taught what anxiety is, using proper vocabulary and explanations. (There is a quick reference provided with the bonus worksheets.)

Be sure to vary the word anxiety to include, fear, nervous, scared, uncomfortable, and uncertainty. Some children will fight the idea that they are anxious but admit to being scared.

If a child has a therapist or supportive parents, this should be happening mostly through one of those paths. For a child who has strong parental and therapeutic support, some of these areas will not need to be addressed by you, but you should be aware of them and make sure that they are part of the support outside of school. The knowledge of anxiety and the skills needed are a must in order for you to create a successful plan for the child. If you notice that parts of what is mentioned below are missing, talk to the parents to make sure the child has these key parts.

However, if this information is not being provided outside of the school, you will need to make sure the child works with the school counselor, whenever possible. The school counselor will need to pull the child and spend some time discussing what anxiety is, how it looks, and what it feels like, why it happens, etc. (Depending on your district, you may have to get permission from parents for a child to visit a counselor within the school.)

Make sure that the school counselor has a strong understanding of anxiety before sending a child to visit. Guidance counselors have an incredibly difficult job within a school and wear many hats as well.

They may not have the educational training or experience in anxiety to be of much help to a child in this area. Make sure that the person educating the child on anxiety has a solid, realistic concept of anxiety.

If a school counselor is not an option, you, as the educator, can spend some one-on-one time with a particular child during study center, lunch, or recess. As you teach the child about anxiety, be sure to reference examples to your life as an adult or a child. Include the language that was shared with you previously in this book, along with the image of the anxiety cycle. It is often easier for a child to connect to an anxious situation that is affecting someone else (either in real life or a character in a book) before connecting the concepts of anxiety to themselves. There are several resources later in the book and on the website that can help a child understand anxiety in general and as it applies to them personally.

As children begin to understand the role anxiety plays in their life, ask them to name some things that they are unhappy about because of anxiety. They may say that they want to attend a birthday party, participate in the school play, share their presentation with the whole class, or play tag on recess with their friends but cannot because of their anxiety. Help them realize that as they work towards managing their anxiety, they will be able to do these things that seem too challenging right now.

Understand the Externalization of Anxiety

An important part of teaching kids to understand and manage their anxiety is to treat anxiety as an external problem. For younger children, you can refer to their anxiety as a worry monster. For older children, you can refer to it as simply a worry or have them create a unique name for their "grown-up" version of a worry monster.

Anxiety is a bully. It bosses the child around, tells them they are not good enough, and causes high amounts of fear. The anxious child begins to see anxiety as a part of them, bringing down their self-confidence and opinion of themselves. The best way to help the child battle anxiety is to name the worry monster, thus, making sure that the anxiety is seen externally. This process allows children to keep their own identify strong while externalizing the anxiety as the bully.

It is important that you explain to the child that the anxious thoughts and feelings are being created by a worry monster or bully. This worry monster or worry bully is trying to scare them but that they do not have to listen to it. This idea separates the anxiety from the identity of the child.

Use fictitious examples of kids who may be mean or bossy at school to illustrate the idea of the worry monster in their head. Just as a child would walk away from the bully at school, and not listen to them, she does not have to listen to the one in her head.

The task of naming the worry monster should be given to the child. There are no guidelines when deciding on a name, simply let the child create a name in which to reference when he is being told false information by the worry monster. Some children select a name tied to anxiety, such as Brain Bully, Brain Monster, Meanie, Mr. Perfect, Mr. Negative, or Amy G. Dala (from the word amygdala). Other children pick names simply because they like the name.

Once the child has named their worry monster, have him draw a picture of what he imagines it looks like. Encourage him to be creative and take his time, adding colors and details. (For older children who may find this silly, ask them to create something through a computer program, with clay, or on canvas.) Have the child keep this somewhere to serve as a reminder that the worry monster is the anxiety, not the child.

Now that the child has a name and an image of this awful worry monster, it is time to start putting the anxiety in its place! When the child begins to feel anxious, you and the child must refer to the worry monster by name rather than talking directly to the child. When you talk to the worry rather than the child, it takes away the negativity the child feels about themselves. You will teach a child how to talk back to their anxiety as part of the anxiety management section of the plan.

Understanding to Expect Worry

As the child begins to understand and apply what she has learned about how anxiety works and externalizing the anxiety with a worry monster, it is time to help her understand to expect anxiety to be present during certain situations throughout the day.

The child should expect the worry to show up and that it is normal and occurs at different times for different reasons. Anxiety showing up is not something to be feared, as she will have the skills to manage the discomfort that may arise. Help children learn to expect the worry rather than to be surprised by it. For children who fear tests, explain that they should expect to feel worried prior to a test. If a child has a hard time separating from a parent in the morning, expect worry to arrive during school drop off. Having the expectation that worry will occur gives them time to plan for how to manage it when it arrives. It also allows you to expect the child to be worried so you can be prepared to support her during this time. Over time, as the child manages the anxiety, the amygdala learns not to respond with a fight or flight approach during this situation.

Acknowledge the Feeling of Anxiety

Early on children are not experienced enough to realize that the thoughts and feelings in their mind and body are a result of anxiety. Through an understanding of how anxiety works and relates to them personally, they will gain a stronger sense of self-awareness. Over time, they will begin to develop the ability to recognize the feelings of anxiety as they arise. They should acknowledge to themselves that there is nothing dangerous happening to them, rather their anxiety is creeping in. By acknowledging this fact, they are able to use their learned skills to manage anxiety and reduce their negative thoughts and feelings in order to meet their goals of school success.

Acknowledge that the Child Knows What to Do

Now that the child has expected the worry, it has arrived with physical and mental symptoms, the child will be able to acknowledge that he can manage the anxiety with the learned skills. This is powerful as the child no longer needs to seek reassurance or avoidance because she has her own skill set to access. The skills may be weak in the beginning, where support is still needed for success, but the child is moving towards creating new habits and independence.

Managing Anxiety with Coping Skills

Steps of Managing Anxiety

You cannot push a child to work through and handle the discomfort of anxiety without the necessary skills. At this point, a child has an understanding of anxiety but needs the skills to manage the anxiety in order to work through uncomfortable situations. This book refers to the necessary skills needed to manage anxiety as coping skills. Coping skills are the tools used to help you handle difficult situations. There are a variety of coping skills that a child can use. A child who receives therapy outside of school should be familiar with this concept. Be sure to ask the child or her parents what her typical coping skills are so that you can include them in the school plan. If a child is not familiar with this idea, you will need to make sure the skills are acquired before he is expected to enter the anxiety-inducing situations. Coping skills should be explained, modeled, and practiced with a child when they are not anxious. As the child learns to use these coping skills, she will utilize them as anxiety arises to move through the challenging thoughts or feelings.

The most common and versatile coping skills are described below. These can be used for nearly every child regardless of their anxieties or age. Like always, they can be easily modified to fit a particular child.

Deep Breaths

The breathing center of the brain is directly tied to higher order brain functions. When anxiety is coursing through the body, the brain has entered the "fight or flight" mode, allowing only survival skills to be accessible. There is no rational thinking occurring during this state of mind. Breathing is not intended to make the anxious feelings go away, rather it allows the mind to re-engage and move into the skills needed to stay and work through the anxiety in a productive way. It is often the first skill to use, as it slows the heart rate and breathing and allows rational thought to return. It can be used to prepare for, or throughout, the anxiety-inducing situation. It does take some practice to breathe effectively. Deep breathing should be practiced many times throughout the day when a child is not anxious.

The box breathing technique is simple for all children. A child will take a deep breath in, filling their stomach, hold for 4 seconds. Then, release that breathe slowly over the course of 4 seconds. Another deep breath should fill the stomach and hold for 4 seconds, followed by a slow release taking 4 seconds. The image below shows a graphic for visual learners. The image can be placed on a child's desk, kept in their pocket, or on a note card to reference during structured breaks. It serves as a reminder, when high anxiety is present, that the first step in managing anxiety should be breathing.

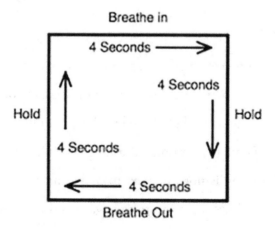

Engage the Five Senses

Similar to deep breathing, this skill is used to slow the heart rate and breathing and re-engage the mind. This can be done along with deep, focused breathing or independently. As the child engages their 5 senses, thoughts and feelings are brought into the present, as a form of mindfulness. The idea is to take slow deep breaths while naming 5 things you see, 4 things you hear, 3 things you can feel, 2 things you can smell, and 1 thing you can taste (when applicable). By breathing slowly and focusing on the senses, anxious thoughts are calmed and the rational part of the brain begins to re-engage. As with the breathing technique, having reminders to use the 5 senses calming technique is critical to children learning to cope with anxiety. There is a poster included with the bonus worksheets that can be used for this technique.

Talking Back to Anxiety

Talking back to the worry uses the externalized worry monster that was previously created. When worry arrives, as expected, the child should make sure that he addresses his worry in the following ways (this can be done aloud or internally depending on the child's comfort level).

Talking back to anxiety is a clear reminder to the child that anxiety is around but that they are in charge. The child is now educated enough to know that even though anxiety feels bad, it cannot hurt him. The child, not the anxiety, holds all of the power. Here are some examples of talking back to anxiety:

- A child with perfectionist tendencies starts to feel anxious over making a mistake. The child says to the worry, "Mr. Perfect, I know you are trying to tell me mistakes are bad but I know that it is ok to make a mistake. I am not going to listen to you." As an educator, you might say, "Mr. Perfect, I see that you are trying to tell [child's name] that he has to be perfect, but we all know that nobody is perfect and that is ok."

- A child with separation anxiety starts to worry when entering school. As an educator, you can say, "It sure looks like Bossy Pants is trying to scare you. I know Bossy Pants is loud and scary but you are brave and know that you will see your parents as soon as school is finished. Be brave and don't listen to mean old Bossy Pants." A child may say, "Bossy Pants is scaring me about school right now. I am telling her that she is just a bully and even though I feel scared, I know I will see my mom and dad after school."

- A teacher notices a child, who has a fear about germs, avoiding the doorknob. The teacher may say, "I see that Meanie is making it hard for you to open the door right now. What can you say to Meanie to make him quiet down?" A child may say, "Leave me alone Meanie. Go pick on someone else. I am going to open this door and go outside."

- For an older child, who may be worried about giving a class presentation, the teacher may say, "I notice the anxiety is trying to convince you that you are not able to speak in front of your peers, but I know that you can because you have a lot of great information to share. Do not listen to the anxiety." A child could reply with, "Yes, the anxiety is trying to talk be out of this but I have worked hard and practiced what I am going to say. I am able to get through this."

Externalizing the anxiety by naming and referring to it as a worry monster, does not make the anxiety disappear, but it separates the anxiety from the child's identity. The more often that the child can reframe her thinking by standing up to the worry monster, talking back to it, and defying what it says, the more success a child will have in lessening the anxiety.

Notecard Reminders

Help the child create a few notecards supporting his goals of managing the anxiety. These notecards can be kept in pockets, on desks, in a backpack, etc. He can then access these reminders as encouragement as he works through facing his anxiety. Each note card should look something like this:

I want to _____, so I will _____.

Example: I want to eat in the cafeteria, so I will bravely sit at the last table for 10 minutes each day this week as I prepare to eat in the cafeteria with my friends.

Similarly, children can create notes of positive self talk, accessing them when needed. Each child will have individual ideas of what should be included on these cards. It can range from, "I have played outside before without being stung by a bee" to "It may feel like everyone is looking at me in the hallway, but they are not actually all watching me as I walk between classes." The wording can also be more generic, such as, "I am a great friend and proud of my writing abilities." The goal is to encourage a child in their moments of weakness. It is important that these reminders of positivity be realistic. For a child who worries about earning high grades on a test, she should not write, "I am so smart and I will get every answer correct." Rather, the positive reminder should be, "I worked really hard to prepare for this test and know that I can do my very best." These reminders can be glued inside of notebooks, stuck in pockets, or written on the inside of hands.

Manageability

The plan and expectations that are created must be manageable by breaking it down into parts. A child with anxiety is easily overwhelmed when working through a difficult situation. In order to help a child gain confidence and independence, she needs to experience moments of success. This can be achieved by breaking down the task or event into smaller parts. As each small step is successfully managed, the child is able to push through the discomfort more successfully.

For a child who is not attending any school, the mere thought of returning to school invokes incredible anxiety. While the ultimate goal is to attend school full time, begin by creating a plan that focuses on attending one class while discussing adding more classes at a later date. The end result is the same, but the way of presenting it is more manageable.

This same idea should be used for all anxieties. The ultimate goal should always be to reduce anxiety from the situation and move forward like a "non-anxious" child. However, it takes a long time to get to that point. Break down the whole into pieces and focus on achieving success in the small parts first. Here are some examples:

- Test anxiety- Have a child work towards completing the first 5 questions independently. Once those 5 questions have been completed, re-evaluate to see if the child needs a structured break to get back on track or if it is possible to continue right away.

- Perfectionism- Encourage a child to write at least three sentences before asking you for assistance. Once those sentences have been completed, re-evaluate to see if the child needs a structured break to get back on track or if it is possible to continue.

- Fear of bees outside- Support the child in standing outside for three minutes with your support. Once those 3 minutes have passed, re-evaluate to see if the child needs a structured break to get back on track or if it is possible to continue.

In addition to breaking tasks down into smaller pieces, middle schoolers and high schoolers can benefit from a well thought out schedule. Create a tween or teen's schedule to include a first period study center which allows the child to come to school and enter a calm, quiet environment where he can get his mind right for the day. Think of the day as two halves, before lunch and after lunch, with lunch occurring as close to the middle of the day as possible. Plan for one or two rigorous core classes before lunch and the remaining core classes after lunch. End the day with the most enjoyable class or less structured elective. This makes the day more manageable as it allows moments of down time in between times of higher intensity.

By experiencing success in small parts, a child's confidence is increased giving him the motivation to continue the hard work of managing his anxiety. It can be slow and tedious, but once again, the time and effort put in now are intended for long term success.

Structured Breaks

The overall goal is for the child to manage the anxiety independently whenever and wherever it arises. This only happens after intense practice and many successes. While the learning process happens, the child will need support that is detailed in the plan. A child who is not able to do the steps of managing anxiety independently will still be doing these same steps with the designated staff member in another location. If a child leaves the classroom, due to anxiety, this would be considered a "structured break". The expectations and set routine for the structured breaks should be clearly laid out within an IEP or 504.

This is important. Be sure that you have a solid understanding of a structured break for children dealing with anxiety. Anxious children may need opportunities to leave the classroom, as they are unable to deal with the discomfort of their anxiety independently or in the confines of the classroom. As part of the plan, you designated support staff members within the school. This is where the child is to go whenever he needs a break. A child should not have to ask permission to take a break, rather the expectations for these breaks must be clearly set ahead of time: Where does the child go for the quiet break? Must an adult accompany her? How long can the break last? What is the expectation in the break location? If the expectations are not followed, what happens? Most children who are using the break for appropriate reasons do not take advantage of these opportunities.

There are two key aspects that must be implemented to make breaks useful for anxious children with the goal of managing anxiety rather than avoidance.

First, the break plan must not simply be quiet, unstructured, free time. The plan must allow breaks where the child works on management skills and returns to class. There should be a location within the school where the child goes to work through the anxiety in an appropriate manner. There is a set routine that occurs while on this break. For example, a child can have a set of notecards to reference where she focuses on her goals for managing anxiety. Similarly, the child can have access to the 5 senses calming technique to lessen the anxiety, with the goal of returning to the location in which he left. Another idea is to role play with the designated support staff. The role play focuses on managing the anxiety around the situation in which the child is struggling.

If a child is simply allowed to leave the room and go to a quiet place and play on a phone, hang out with an adult, or sit quietly in a bean bag chair, there is no reason a child would stay in class when feeling anxious. Also, children who leave the classroom repeatedly and for long durations, begin to get anxious about returning to class in front of their peers and falling behind in the classwork that was missed while they were out of the room. The structured break should only last for a designated time (5-10 minutes), can only be used to work through the anxiety as laid out in the plan, and should have every adult involved on the same page.

Second, there should be a weaning off process in place, allowing the child to manage the anxiety in the classroom rather than leaving frequently. The weaning off process should be mentioned in the management section of the plan. The goal is to help the child use the skills, with adult support in the beginning, while getting to the point that the skills can be used independently within the classroom.

Key Points Necessary for A Child's Successful Management of School Anxiety

- The goal is not to remove anxiety, rather retraining the amygdala to function in times of true danger as it was intended.

- Anxiety is normal, until it becomes a problem and interferes in daily life.

- Anxiety is a cycle that needs to be fixed to function properly.

- An understanding of how a child's anxiety is currently affecting him and what the symptoms are.

- Anxiety needs to be externalized.

- Why the child wants to retrain their brain and manage anxiety.

- Understands the coping skills needed to move into the anxiety such as breathing and talking back to the anxiety.

- Their goal is to move into the anxiety and use the skills learned which creates new positive habits and retrains the brain.

Consistency is Key for Success

Consistency and structure within a classroom are mandatory for all children to be successful. This same idea applies to the plan you create. Every person, at home and at school, must support and implement the plan as it was designed. Anxious children are always looking for an "easy" way out and if they find a "weak" spot, they will take it. This is because avoidance feels much better, in the moment than working through the anxiety. Within the school, the classroom teacher(s), nurse, elective teachers, support staff, cafeteria aides, etc. must all be aware of the plan and the language used within the plan. If the plan dictates that a child not visit the nurse for anxiety, then no adult should allow the child to visit the nurse. With structured breaks, the child must be held accountable by the adult to use the breaks as designed. This plan must be honored with consistency, validity, and authenticity or you will not get the results you are seeking, which is unfair to the child and the teacher.

Now What?

Phew...that was a lot of information. You now have a foundational understanding of anxiety and the impact it can have on a child while at school. All children deserve to attend school where they are successful...academically, emotionally, and mentally. Sadly, anxiety rips these expected comforts away from the child and their family. I personally want to thank you for taking the time to read through this, as you are one step closer to making an incredibly positive difference in a child's life.

From this point on, with your completed exercises and gathered data, you can form a team, create a plan, and implement the strategies to meet the goal of supporting a child as she works towards independent anxiety management in the school setting. I am always available to do what I can to help you with individual children in your school. I can be reached at goodbyeanxietyhellojoy@gmail.com. I personally answer every email, doing my best to offer support.

Once parents and educators work together with the goal of making sure that the child has the necessary skills for success, combined with the proper understanding and support from the adults in their life, there is no stopping them! With anxiety well managed at school, home life improves as well. Suddenly, the anxious, clingy, needy child is laughing with friends, gaining confidence in themselves, and enjoying life. And you can sleep each night knowing you did your part in ensuring that each and every child is able to live their best life!

Resources

To access the printable PDFs of all of the exercises and images in this book, as well as the additional bonus printables, go to https://goodbyeanxietyhellojoy.com/freeprintables and enter the password *iboughtthebook.*

Examples of (non-academic) IEP goals for managing anxiety at school

IEP goals aimed at improving anxiety mandate that the school/staff provide tools, support and assessments with the intention of improving anxiety in the school setting. These goals should be in addition to academic goals when necessary.

- When facing a challenging situation, [Child's Name] will define the problem and come up with at least two possible solutions to the problem % of the time.
- When needing assistance, [Child's Name] will demonstrate appropriate skills in asking for help at appropriate times % of the time.
- When help is needed, [Child's Name] will explain the kind of help needed for a situation % of the time.

- When negative feelings or behaviors arise, [Child's Name] will attend a structured break held at an appropriate time and place where [Child's Name]t will try to identify triggers and possible strategies for improvement % of the time.

- When given a task that [Child's Name] correctly identifies as difficult, [Child's Name] will create a plan for accomplishing the task % of the time.

- [Child's Name] will increase independent work time by completing one task with one or less adult prompts 3 out of 5 opportunities to do so.

- [Child's Name] will transition independently from class to class % of the time by the end of the second semester.

- [Child's Name] will stay in class for the entire period % of the time by the end of the first semester.

Literature Recommendations for Normalizing and Discussing Anxiety

The Owl Who Was Afraid of the Dark by Jill Tomlinson and Paul Howard (Ages 4 and up)

Begin at the Beginning: A Little Artist Learns about Life by Amy Schwartz (Ages 4 and up)

Something Might Happen by Helen Lester, ill. by Lynn Musinger (Ages 4 and up)

Wanda's Monster by Eileen Spinelli, ill. by Nancy Hayashi (Ages 4 and up)

The Opposite by Tom MacRae and Elena Odriozola (Ages 4 and up)

William, the What-If Wonder: On His First Day of School by Carol Wulff (Ages 4 and up)

The OK Book by Amy Krouse Rosenthal and Tom Lichtenheld (Ages 4 and up)

Beautiful Oops! By Barney Saltzberg (Ages 4 and up)

Spaghetti in a Hot Dog Bun by Kathy Hiatt (Ages 4 and up)

I am Human by Susan Verde (Ages 4 and up)

Your Fantastic Elastic Brain: Stretch It, Shape It by JoAnn Deak, Ph.D. and Sarah Ackerley (Ages 4 and up)

The Humphrey Book Series by Betty Birney (Ages 8 and up)

So B. It by Sarah Weeks (Ages 8 and up)

The Unteachables by Gordon Korman (Ages 8 and up)

Counting by 7's by Holly Goldberg Sloan (Ages 10 and up)

Fish in a Tree by Lynda Mullaly Hunt (Ages 10 and up)

Finding Audrey by Sophie Kinsella (Ages 12 and up)

What To Say Next by Julia Buxbaum (Ages 12 and up)

A Quiet Kind of Thunder by Sara Barnard (Ages 14 and up)

It's Kind of a Funny Story by Ned Vizzini (Ages 14 and up)

Eleanor And Park by Rainbow Powell (Ages 14 and up)

The Upside of Unrequited by Becky Albertalli (Ages 14 and up)

Fangirl by Rainbow Powell (Ages 14 and up)

Turtles All the Way Down by John Green (Ages 14 and up)

Obsessed: A Memoir of My Life with OCD by Allison Britz (Ages 14 and up)